FAST FEAST REPEAT RECIPES

COOKBOOK

A Comprehensive Guide to Intermittent Fasting, Delicious Recipes, and Sustainable Lifestyle Changes for Fast Results and Long-Term Success.

MICHAEL JUNIOR

Copyright © 2023 by Michael Junior

CONTENT

INTRODUCTION 4

Cucumber and Tuna Salad 5

Quinoa and Black Bean Bowl 8

Turkey Lettuce Wraps 11

Eggplant and Tomato Casserole 14

Chickpea and Vegetable Curry 17

Spinach and Feta Stuffed Chicken Breast .. 20

Baked Cod with Lemon and Herbs 23

Lentil Soup 26

Sweet Potato and Black Bean Salad 29

Chicken and Vegetable Skewers 32

Caprese Salad 35

Greek Yogurt Parfait 38

Cauliflower Rice Stir-Fry 41

Turkey and Quinoa Stuffed Peppers 44

Mushroom and Spinach Omelet 47

Salmon and Asparagus Foil Packets 50

Vegetarian Stir-Fry 53

Grilled Chicken and Quinoa Bowl 56

Avocado and Egg Salad 59

Green Smoothie Bowl 62

CONCLUSION 65

INTRODUCTION

Welcome to a culinary adventure that goes beyond recipes, enabling you to embrace an empowered and well-being lifestyle. We go on a novel investigation of Intermittent Fasting in the domain of 'Fast Feast Repeat,' where every meal becomes a celebration of attentive feeding.

This cookbook is more than simply a collection of recipes; it's a guide to regaining control of your health, appreciating wonderful flavors, and experiencing the joy of balanced living again and again.

Join us as we start on a gastronomic adventure that promises not only quick results but also a feast of energy, which will be repeated with each delectable, health-infused dish.

Cucumber and Tuna Salad

Scenario:
Imagine a refreshing and satisfying salad that combines the crispness of cucumbers with the protein-packed goodness of tuna. This Cucumber and Tuna Salad is not only a breeze to prepare but also a delightful way to enjoy a light, nutrient-rich meal.

Ingredients:
- 1 large cucumber, thinly sliced
- 1 can of tuna in water, drained
- 1 cup cherry tomatoes, halved
- 1/4 cup Kalamata olives, pitted and sliced
- 2 tablespoons red onion, finely chopped
- 2 tablespoons feta cheese, crumbled (optional)
- 2 tablespoons extra-virgin olive oil
- 1 tablespoon lemon juice
- Salt and pepper to taste
- Fresh parsley for garnish

Preparation:
1. In a large bowl, combine the sliced cucumber, drained tuna, halved cherry tomatoes, sliced olives, chopped red onion, and crumbled feta cheese (if using).

2. In a small bowl, whisk together the extra-virgin olive oil and lemon juice. Season with salt and pepper to taste.
3. Drizzle the dressing over the cucumber and tuna mixture. Gently toss the salad until all ingredients are well coated.
4. Allow the salad to marinate for a few minutes to let the flavors meld together.
5. Garnish with fresh parsley just before serving.

Benefits:
- **Rich in Protein:** Tuna provides a high-quality protein source, which is essential for muscle repair and overall body function.
- **Hydrating and Low-Calorie:** Cucumbers are mostly water, contributing to hydration, and they are low in calories, making this salad a great choice for those looking to maintain or lose weight.
- **Packed with Vitamins and Minerals:** Cherry tomatoes offer vitamins like C and K, while olives provide healthy fats and antioxidants.

Application:
- **Lunch on the Go:** Pack this salad in a sealed container for a convenient and healthy lunch option. The crisp texture of

the cucumber will hold up well, and the flavors will intensify over time.

- **Light Dinner Option:** Serve this salad as a light and refreshing dinner, especially on warm evenings when a heavy meal might not be as appealing.
- **Side Dish at Gatherings:** Make a larger batch to serve as a colorful and flavorful side dish at barbecues, picnics, or potluck gatherings.

This Cucumber and Tuna Salad is a versatile dish that caters to those seeking a quick and nutritious option, without compromising on taste and satisfaction. Enjoy the benefits of a well-balanced meal with this simple yet delicious recipe.

Quinoa and Black Bean Bowl

Scenario:
Imagine a wholesome and flavorful bowl that brings together the nutty goodness of quinoa and the protein punch of black beans. This Quinoa and Black Bean Bowl is not only a culinary delight but also a nutritious powerhouse that fuels your body with essential nutrients.

Ingredients:
- 1 cup quinoa, rinsed
- 2 cups black beans, cooked and drained
- 1 cup corn kernels (fresh or frozen)
- 1 cup cherry tomatoes, quartered
- 1/4 cup red onion, finely chopped
- 1/4 cup fresh cilantro, chopped
- Juice of 1 lime
- 2 tablespoons olive oil
- 1 teaspoon ground cumin
- Salt and pepper to taste
- Avocado slices for garnish (optional)

Preparation:
1. Cook quinoa according to package instructions. Fluff with a fork and let it cool to room temperature.
2. In a large bowl, combine the cooked quinoa, black beans, corn, cherry

tomatoes, red onion, and chopped cilantro.
3. In a small bowl, whisk together lime juice, olive oil, ground cumin, salt, and pepper.
4. Drizzle the dressing over the quinoa and black bean mixture. Gently toss until all ingredients are evenly coated.
5. Allow the bowl to sit for a few minutes to let the flavors meld together.
6. Garnish with avocado slices just before serving.

Benefits:
- **Protein Powerhouse:** Both quinoa and black beans are excellent sources of plant-based protein, making this bowl ideal for vegetarians and those looking to incorporate more protein into their diet.
- **Rich in Fiber:** Black beans and quinoa are high in fiber, promoting digestive health and providing a sense of fullness.
- **Loaded with Vitamins and Minerals:** The variety of colorful vegetables in this bowl ensures a good mix of vitamins, minerals, and antioxidants.

Application:
- **Meal Prep:** Prepare a batch of Quinoa and Black Bean Bowls at the beginning of the week for quick and convenient lunches or dinners.

- **Vegetarian Main Course:** Serve this dish as a satisfying and nutritious main course for vegetarian meals.
- **Side Dish at Potlucks:** Bring this bowl to potluck gatherings as a flavorful and nutritious side dish that complements a variety of main courses.

This Quinoa and Black Bean Bowl is a versatile and healthful option for those seeking a well-rounded meal that's not only delicious but also packed with essential nutrients. Enjoy the vibrant colors and flavors while nourishing your body with this wholesome bowl.

Turkey Lettuce Wraps

Scenario:

Picture a meal that's light, flavorful, and delightfully hands-on. These Turkey Lettuce Wraps offer a tasty and healthy alternative to traditional wraps. Packed with lean protein and fresh ingredients, they make for a satisfying and low-carb option for any meal.

Ingredients:

- 1 pound ground turkey
- 1 tablespoon olive oil
- 1 small onion, finely chopped
- 2 cloves garlic, minced
- 1 teaspoon ground cumin
- 1 teaspoon chili powder
- 1/2 teaspoon paprika
- Salt and pepper to taste
- Iceberg or butter lettuce leaves, washed and separated
- 1 cup cherry tomatoes, diced
- 1 avocado, diced
- 1/4 cup fresh cilantro, chopped
- Greek yogurt or sour cream for serving (optional)

Preparation:

1. Heat olive oil in a skillet over medium heat. Add chopped onions and garlic, sauté until softened.

2. Add ground turkey to the skillet, breaking it apart with a spoon. Cook until browned.
3. Stir in ground cumin, chili powder, paprika, salt, and pepper. Allow the spices to coat the turkey evenly. Cook for an additional 2-3 minutes.
4. Remove the skillet from heat. Arrange lettuce leaves on a serving platter.
5. Spoon the seasoned turkey mixture onto each lettuce leaf.
6. Top with diced cherry tomatoes, avocado, and fresh cilantro.
7. Optionally, drizzle with Greek yogurt or sour cream for added creaminess.
8. Serve immediately, allowing everyone to assemble their own wraps at the table.

Benefits:
- **Lean Protein:** Turkey is a lean source of protein, promoting muscle health and providing a sense of satiety.
- **Low-Carb Option:** Substituting lettuce for traditional wraps reduces the carb content, making it suitable for those following low-carb or keto diets.
- **Nutrient-Rich:** The inclusion of vegetables like tomatoes and avocado adds essential vitamins, minerals, and healthy fats.

Application:
- **Quick Weeknight Dinner:** These Turkey Lettuce Wraps are perfect for a quick and healthy weeknight dinner that's both delicious and satisfying.
- **Lunchbox Option:** Prepare the turkey mixture in advance and assemble the wraps just before eating for a convenient and portable lunch option.
- **Appetizer at Gatherings:** Serve these wraps as a healthy and interactive appetizer at gatherings or parties.

These Turkey Lettuce Wraps are a flavorful and nutritious alternative to traditional wraps, offering a burst of freshness and a satisfying combination of textures. Enjoy the convenience and health benefits of this delightful dish.

Eggplant and Tomato Casserole

Scenario:

Imagine a comforting casserole that melds the earthy richness of eggplant with the vibrant flavors of tomatoes. This Eggplant and Tomato Casserole is a hearty, yet healthy dish that celebrates the goodness of fresh produce and is perfect for a cozy family dinner.

Ingredients:

- 2 large eggplants, thinly sliced
- 4 large tomatoes, sliced
- 3 cloves garlic, minced
- 1/2 cup grated Parmesan cheese
- 1/4 cup fresh basil, chopped
- 1/4 cup fresh parsley, chopped
- 2 tablespoons olive oil
- Salt and pepper to taste
- 1 cup mozzarella cheese, shredded (optional, for topping)

Preparation:

1. Preheat the oven to 375°F (190°C). Grease a baking dish with olive oil.
2. Arrange a layer of eggplant slices at the bottom of the baking dish. Sprinkle with minced garlic, salt, and pepper.

3. Place a layer of tomato slices over the eggplant. Drizzle with olive oil and sprinkle with half of the Parmesan cheese, basil, and parsley.
4. Repeat the layers, finishing with a final layer of eggplant on top. Drizzle with olive oil and sprinkle the remaining Parmesan, basil, and parsley.
5. Optionally, sprinkle mozzarella cheese over the top for a gooey, melted finish.
6. Cover the baking dish with foil and bake for 30 minutes. Remove the foil and bake for an additional 15-20 minutes or until the top is golden and bubbly.
7. Let the casserole rest for a few minutes before serving.

Benefits:
- **Rich in Antioxidants:** Tomatoes and eggplants are loaded with antioxidants, supporting overall health and well-being.
- **Low-Calorie Option:** This casserole is a lower-calorie alternative to many traditional casseroles, making it suitable for those watching their calorie intake.
- **Source of Essential Nutrients:** Eggplant provides dietary fiber, while tomatoes contribute vitamins A and C.

Application:

- **Vegetarian Main Course:** Serve this Eggplant and Tomato Casserole as a wholesome vegetarian main course, accompanied by a side salad or crusty bread.
- **Side Dish at Potlucks:** Bring this casserole to potluck gatherings as a flavorful and nutrient-rich side dish that pairs well with various main courses.
- **Make-Ahead Dinner:** Prepare the casserole ahead of time and refrigerate until ready to bake for a convenient make-ahead dinner option.

This Eggplant and Tomato Casserole is a delightful way to savor the flavors of the Mediterranean while enjoying the health benefits of fresh vegetables. It's a versatile dish that's sure to become a family favorite.

Chickpea and Vegetable Curry

Scenario:
Experience the aromatic allure of a wholesome curry that combines the protein-packed goodness of chickpeas with an array of vibrant vegetables.

This Chickpea and Vegetable Curry is a celebration of spices and flavors, creating a satisfying and nourishing dish that's perfect for a hearty dinner.

Ingredients:
- 2 cans (15 oz each) chickpeas, drained and rinsed
- 1 large onion, finely chopped
- 3 cloves garlic, minced
- 1 tablespoon ginger, grated
- 1 large carrot, diced
- 1 bell pepper, diced
- 1 zucchini, diced
- 1 cup cauliflower florets
- 1 can (14 oz) diced tomatoes
- 1 can (14 oz) coconut milk
- 2 tablespoons curry powder
- 1 teaspoon ground cumin
- 1 teaspoon ground coriander
- 1/2 teaspoon turmeric
- Salt and pepper to taste
- Fresh cilantro for garnish

- Cooked rice or naan for serving

Preparation:

1. In a large pot, heat a bit of oil over medium heat. Add chopped onions and cook until softened.
2. Add minced garlic and grated ginger, sauté for another minute until fragrant.
3. Stir in curry powder, ground cumin, ground coriander, and turmeric. Cook for 1-2 minutes until the spices are toasted.
4. Add diced carrots, bell pepper, zucchini, and cauliflower to the pot. Stir to coat the vegetables with the spice mixture.
5. Pour in the diced tomatoes with their juice and coconut milk. Bring the mixture to a gentle simmer.
6. Add the chickpeas to the pot, season with salt and pepper, and let the curry simmer for 20-25 minutes until the vegetables are tender.
7. Adjust the seasoning to taste and serve the curry over cooked rice or with naan.
8. Garnish with fresh cilantro before serving.

Benefits:

- **Plant-Based Protein:** Chickpeas are a great source of plant-based protein, making this curry a satisfying meatless option.

- **Nutrient-Rich Vegetables:** The variety of vegetables provides essential vitamins, minerals, and fiber.
- **Anti-Inflammatory Spices:** Turmeric, cumin, and coriander are known for their anti-inflammatory properties.

Application:

- **Meatless Monday Dinner:** This Chickpea and Vegetable Curry is an excellent choice for a flavorful and filling meatless Monday dinner.
- **Batch Cooking for Meal Prep:** Make a large batch and store it in portions for easy meal prep throughout the week.
- **Serve at Gatherings:** Impress your guests by serving this hearty and aromatic curry at gatherings or potluck dinners.

Enjoy the aromatic symphony of spices and the richness of chickpeas and vegetables with this Chickpea and Vegetable Curry. It's a versatile dish that caters to both vegetarians and those looking to incorporate more plant-based meals into their diet.

Spinach and Feta Stuffed Chicken Breast

Scenario:

Elevate your weeknight dinner with a gourmet touch. Imagine succulent chicken breasts filled with a savory blend of spinach and feta, creating a dish that's not only visually impressive but also bursting with flavors.

These Spinach and Feta Stuffed Chicken Breasts are a delicious treat for a special dinner at home.

Ingredients:

- 4 boneless, skinless chicken breasts
- 2 cups fresh spinach, chopped
- 1 cup feta cheese, crumbled
- 1/4 cup sun-dried tomatoes, chopped (optional)
- 2 cloves garlic, minced
- 1 tablespoon olive oil
- 1 teaspoon dried oregano
- Salt and pepper to taste
- Toothpicks or kitchen twine for securing

Preparation:

1. Preheat the oven to 375°F (190°C).

2. In a skillet, heat olive oil over medium heat. Add minced garlic and sauté until fragrant.
3. Add chopped spinach to the skillet and cook until wilted. Remove from heat and let it cool.
4. In a mixing bowl, combine the wilted spinach, crumbled feta, sun-dried tomatoes (if using), dried oregano, salt, and pepper. Mix well.
5. Butterfly each chicken breast by slicing horizontally, leaving one edge intact. Open the chicken like a book.
6. Spoon the spinach and feta mixture onto one side of each chicken breast.
7. Close the chicken breast over the filling and secure with toothpicks or tie with kitchen twine.
8. Place the stuffed chicken breasts in a baking dish. Season the outside with additional salt, pepper, and oregano.
9. Bake in the preheated oven for 25-30 minutes or until the chicken is cooked through.
10. Allow the chicken to rest for a few minutes before slicing.

Benefits:
- **High Protein:** Chicken breast is a lean source of protein, essential for muscle development and repair.

- **Nutrient-Rich Spinach:** Spinach provides a wealth of vitamins, minerals, and antioxidants.
- **Calcium from Feta:** Feta cheese adds a creamy texture and contributes to the dish's calcium content.

Application:
- **Date Night Dinner:** Impress your loved ones with a restaurant-worthy dish perfect for a cozy date night at home.
- **Special Occasion Meal:** Serve these stuffed chicken breasts for special occasions or celebrations.
- **Dinner Party Entree:** Wow your guests by presenting these elegant stuffed chicken breasts as the main course at a dinner party.

These Spinach and Feta Stuffed Chicken Breasts are a delightful combination of flavors and textures, creating a dish that's both comforting and sophisticated. Enjoy the indulgence of a gourmet meal in the comfort of your own home.

Baked Cod with Lemon and Herbs

Scenario:

Transport yourself to the coastal bliss of a Mediterranean dinner with this Baked Cod with Lemon and Herbs. Imagine tender cod fillets infused with the brightness of lemon and the aromatic notes of fresh herbs, creating a dish that's both light and flavorful.

Ingredients:

- 4 cod fillets
- Zest and juice of 1 lemon
- 2 tablespoons fresh parsley, chopped
- 1 tablespoon fresh dill, chopped
- 2 cloves garlic, minced
- 3 tablespoons olive oil
- Salt and pepper to taste
- Lemon slices for garnish

Preparation:

1. Preheat the oven to 400°F (200°C).
2. Pat the cod fillets dry with paper towels and place them in a baking dish.
3. In a small bowl, mix together lemon zest, lemon juice, chopped parsley, chopped dill, minced garlic, olive oil, salt, and pepper.

4. Pour the lemon and herb mixture over the cod fillets, ensuring they are evenly coated.
5. Allow the cod to marinate in the refrigerator for at least 15 minutes to let the flavors infuse.
6. Bake the cod in the preheated oven for 15-20 minutes or until the fish flakes easily with a fork.
7. Garnish with lemon slices before serving.

Benefits:
- **Lean Protein:** Cod is a low-fat, high-protein fish that supports muscle health.
- **Omega-3 Fatty Acids:** Cod is a good source of omega-3 fatty acids, promoting heart health.
- **Antioxidant-Rich Herbs:** Fresh herbs like parsley and dill add not only flavor but also antioxidants to the dish.

Application:
- **Healthy Weeknight Dinner:** Prepare this baked cod for a quick and healthy weeknight dinner that's both delicious and light.
- **Entertaining Guests:** Impress your guests by serving this elegant dish at dinner parties or gatherings.

- **Lunch Option:** Cold leftovers of this baked cod can be flaked over a salad for a refreshing and nutritious lunch.

This Baked Cod with Lemon and Herbs offers a simple yet elegant way to enjoy the delicate flavors of fish enhanced by the zesty brightness of lemon and the aromatic touch of fresh herbs. It's a dish that embodies the essence of Mediterranean cuisine.

Lentil Soup

Scenario:

Imagine a warm bowl of hearty lentil soup, simmering on the stove, filling your kitchen with comforting aromas. This Lentil Soup is a nourishing and flavorful dish that not only warms the soul but also provides a healthy dose of plant-based goodness.

Ingredients:

- 1 cup dry green or brown lentils, rinsed
- 1 onion, finely chopped
- 2 carrots, diced
- 2 celery stalks, diced
- 3 cloves garlic, minced
- 1 can (14 oz) diced tomatoes
- 6 cups vegetable broth
- 1 teaspoon ground cumin
- 1 teaspoon ground coriander
- 1/2 teaspoon smoked paprika
- 1 bay leaf
- Salt and pepper to taste
- 2 tablespoons olive oil
- Fresh parsley for garnish
- Lemon wedges for serving

Preparation:

1. In a large pot, heat olive oil over medium heat. Add chopped onion, carrots, and

celery. Cook until vegetables are softened.

2. Add minced garlic, ground cumin, ground coriander, and smoked paprika. Stir and cook for an additional 2 minutes until fragrant.
3. Pour in the rinsed lentils, diced tomatoes (with their juice), and vegetable broth. Add the bay leaf. Season with salt and pepper to taste.
4. Bring the soup to a boil, then reduce the heat to low. Cover and simmer for 25-30 minutes or until the lentils are tender.
5. Remove the bay leaf and discard. Adjust the seasoning if necessary.
6. Serve the lentil soup hot, garnished with fresh parsley and accompanied by lemon wedges.

Benefits:
- **Rich in Fiber:** Lentils are an excellent source of fiber, promoting digestive health and providing a sense of fullness.
- **Plant-Based Protein:** Lentils are a great plant-based protein source, making this soup suitable for vegetarians and vegans.
- **Nutrient-Dense:** The combination of vegetables and lentils provides a wide range of essential vitamins and minerals.

Application:

- **Meal Prep Staple:** Prepare a batch of lentil soup at the beginning of the week for a quick and nutritious go-to meal.
- **Light Lunch Option:** Enjoy a bowl of lentil soup for a satisfying and light lunch.
- **Starter for Dinners:** Serve this soup as a flavorful and nutritious starter before a main course for family dinners or gatherings.

This Lentil Soup is a comforting and versatile dish that not only satisfies your taste buds but also nourishes your body with essential nutrients. Whether enjoyed on a chilly day or as a wholesome meal option, it's a classic that never fails to deliver warmth and goodness.

Sweet Potato and Black Bean Salad

Scenario:
Envision a vibrant salad that combines the natural sweetness of roasted sweet potatoes with the protein and fiber richness of black beans.

This Sweet Potato and Black Bean Salad is not just a burst of colors on your plate; it's a flavorful and nutrient-packed dish that celebrates wholesome ingredients.

Ingredients:
- 2 large sweet potatoes, peeled and diced
- 1 can (15 oz) black beans, drained and rinsed
- 1 red bell pepper, diced
- 1/2 red onion, finely chopped
- 1/4 cup fresh cilantro, chopped
- Juice of 2 limes
- 3 tablespoons olive oil
- 1 teaspoon ground cumin
- 1 teaspoon chili powder
- Salt and pepper to taste
- Optional: Avocado slices for garnish

Preparation:
1. Preheat the oven to 400°F (200°C).

2. Toss the diced sweet potatoes with 1 tablespoon of olive oil, ground cumin, chili powder, salt, and pepper.
3. Spread the seasoned sweet potatoes in a single layer on a baking sheet. Roast in the preheated oven for 20-25 minutes or until tender and slightly caramelized.
4. In a large bowl, combine the roasted sweet potatoes, black beans, diced red bell pepper, chopped red onion, and cilantro.
5. In a small bowl, whisk together the lime juice and remaining 2 tablespoons of olive oil. Season with salt and pepper.
6. Drizzle the lime dressing over the salad and toss gently to combine.
7. Allow the flavors to meld for a few minutes before serving.
8. Garnish with avocado slices if desired.

Benefits:
- **Rich in Vitamins:** Sweet potatoes provide a wealth of vitamins, including A and C.
- **Plant-Based Protein:** Black beans offer a healthy dose of plant-based protein and fiber.
- **Heart-Healthy Fats:** Olive oil and avocados contribute heart-healthy monounsaturated fats.

Application:
- **Healthy Side Dish:** Serve this salad as a nutritious side dish alongside grilled chicken, fish, or tofu.
- **Light Lunch Option:** Enjoy a satisfying and colorful lunch by topping the salad with grilled shrimp or chickpeas.
- **Potluck Favorite:** Bring this Sweet Potato and Black Bean Salad to potluck gatherings or picnics for a crowd-pleasing and nutritious option.

This Sweet Potato and Black Bean Salad is a delightful fusion of flavors and textures that brings together the earthiness of sweet potatoes, the heartiness of black beans, and the freshness of vegetables.

It's a versatile dish that's perfect for various occasions, from family dinners to social gatherings.

Chicken and Vegetable Skewers

Scenario:

Picture a backyard barbecue with the sizzle of skewers on the grill, releasing a mouthwatering aroma. These Chicken and Vegetable Skewers are a perfect embodiment of summer grilling – a flavorful combination of tender chicken and vibrant vegetables, creating a feast for your senses.

Ingredients:
- 1.5 lbs boneless, skinless chicken breasts, cut into cubes
- 1 red bell pepper, cut into chunks
- 1 yellow bell pepper, cut into chunks
- 1 red onion, cut into chunks
- Cherry tomatoes
- 1 zucchini, sliced
- 3 tablespoons olive oil
- 3 cloves garlic, minced
- 1 teaspoon dried oregano
- 1 teaspoon smoked paprika
- Salt and pepper to taste
- Wooden or metal skewers

Preparation:
1. If using wooden skewers, soak them in water for at least 30 minutes to prevent burning during grilling.

2. In a bowl, combine olive oil, minced garlic, dried oregano, smoked paprika, salt, and pepper to create the marinade.
3. Thread the chicken, bell peppers, red onion, cherry tomatoes, and zucchini onto the skewers, alternating the ingredients.
4. Brush the skewers generously with the marinade, ensuring even coverage.
5. Preheat the grill to medium-high heat.
6. Grill the skewers for 12-15 minutes, turning occasionally, until the chicken is cooked through and the vegetables are charred and tender.
7. Optional: Brush the skewers with additional marinade during grilling for extra flavor.
8. Remove from the grill and let them rest for a few minutes.
9. Serve the Chicken and Vegetable Skewers hot, garnished with fresh herbs if desired.

Benefits:
- **Lean Protein:** Chicken breast provides a lean source of protein for muscle health.
- **Vitamins and Antioxidants:** Bell peppers and tomatoes contribute vitamins A and C, while zucchini adds antioxidants.
- **Heart-Healthy Fats:** Olive oil offers monounsaturated fats that are good for heart health.

Application:

- **Backyard BBQ:** These skewers are a perfect addition to any summer barbecue or outdoor gathering.
- **Family Dinner:** Serve the skewers over a bed of rice or quinoa for a wholesome family dinner.
- **Appetizer for Parties:** Make mini skewers for appetizers at parties or events.

These Chicken and Vegetable Skewers are a delightful and healthy grilling option that brings together the succulence of chicken with the vibrant colors and flavors of assorted vegetables. Perfect for sharing and enjoying the best of summer.

Caprese Salad

Scenario:
Imagine a light and refreshing salad that captures the essence of Italian flavors. The Caprese Salad is a timeless classic that celebrates the simplicity of fresh ingredients.

Picture a vibrant platter adorned with ripe tomatoes, creamy mozzarella, and fragrant basil, drizzled with the finest olive oil – a true symphony of flavors.

Ingredients:
- 4 large tomatoes, sliced
- 1 pound fresh mozzarella cheese, sliced
- Fresh basil leaves
- Extra-virgin olive oil
- Balsamic glaze
- Salt and pepper to taste

Preparation:
1. Arrange the slices of tomatoes and mozzarella alternately on a serving platter.
2. Tuck fresh basil leaves between the tomato and mozzarella slices.
3. Drizzle extra-virgin olive oil generously over the salad.
4. Sprinkle salt and pepper to taste.

5. Finish by drizzling balsamic glaze over the top.
6. Serve the Caprese Salad immediately to preserve the freshness of the ingredients.

Benefits:
- **Rich in Antioxidants:** Tomatoes and basil are packed with antioxidants that contribute to overall health.
- **Source of Calcium and Protein:** Mozzarella provides calcium and protein, essential for bone health and muscle function.
- **Healthy Fats:** Extra-virgin olive oil contributes heart-healthy monounsaturated fats.

Application:
- **Appetizer at Dinners:** Serve as a light and elegant appetizer before a dinner party.
- **Summer Picnic Dish:** Pack individual portions for a refreshing salad to enjoy at picnics or outdoor gatherings.
- **Side Dish for Grilled Meats:** Pair with grilled chicken or steak for a flavorful and balanced meal.

This Caprese Salad is a celebration of simplicity and quality ingredients. Its versatility makes it a go-to option for various occasions, adding a touch of sophistication to any meal. Enjoy the harmony of flavors in every bite.

Greek Yogurt Parfait

Scenario:
Envision a delightful and wholesome breakfast or snack that not only tantalizes your taste buds but also provides a boost of nutrition.

The Greek Yogurt Parfait is a layered masterpiece, combining the creaminess of yogurt with the sweetness of fruits and the crunch of granola, creating a symphony of textures and flavors.

Ingredients:
- 2 cups Greek yogurt (plain or flavored)
- 1 cup mixed berries (strawberries, blueberries, raspberries)
- 1/2 cup granola
- 2 tablespoons honey or maple syrup
- 1/4 cup nuts (almonds, walnuts, or your choice), chopped
- Fresh mint leaves for garnish (optional)

Preparation:
1. In a glass or a bowl, spoon a layer of Greek yogurt to create the base.
2. Add a layer of mixed berries on top of the yogurt.
3. Sprinkle a layer of granola over the berries, providing a satisfying crunch.

4. Drizzle honey or maple syrup over the granola for added sweetness.
5. Repeat the layers until you reach the top of the glass or bowl.
6. Finish with a dollop of Greek yogurt, a few extra berries, and a sprinkle of chopped nuts.
7. Garnish with fresh mint leaves if desired.
8. Serve the Greek Yogurt Parfait immediately to enjoy the contrast of textures.

Benefits:

- **Protein-Packed:** Greek yogurt is rich in protein, aiding in muscle repair and promoting a feeling of fullness.
- **Antioxidant-Rich Berries:** Berries are loaded with antioxidants, contributing to overall health and well-being.
- **Energy from Granola:** Granola provides complex carbohydrates for sustained energy throughout the day.
- **Heart-Healthy Fats:** Nuts offer healthy fats that support heart health.

Application:

- **Quick Breakfast Option:** Assemble this parfait for a quick and nutritious breakfast that requires minimal preparation.

- **Snack for Energy Boost:** Enjoy as a satisfying and energizing snack in the afternoon.
- **Dessert Alternative:** Serve as a healthier dessert option at the end of a meal.

The Greek Yogurt Parfait is not only a treat for your taste buds but also a nutritious and versatile option suitable for various occasions throughout the day. Customize the layers to suit your preferences and dietary needs.

Cauliflower Rice Stir-Fry

Scenario:
Imagine a colorful and flavorful stir-fry that's not only delicious but also low in carbs. The Cauliflower Rice Stir-Fry is a creative and nutritious twist on the classic, using cauliflower rice as a base for a vibrant mix of vegetables and protein, creating a wholesome and satisfying meal.

Ingredients:
- 1 medium-sized cauliflower, riced
- 1 cup broccoli florets
- 1 carrot, julienned
- 1 bell pepper (any color), thinly sliced
- 1 cup snap peas, trimmed
- 2 tablespoons soy sauce or tamari
- 1 tablespoon sesame oil
- 1 tablespoon olive oil
- 3 cloves garlic, minced
- 1 tablespoon ginger, grated
- 1 cup cooked protein of your choice (chicken, shrimp, tofu, etc.)
- Green onions and sesame seeds for garnish
- Salt and pepper to taste

Preparation:
1. Trim the leaves and stem from the cauliflower and cut it into florets. Place the

florets in a food processor and pulse until it resembles rice.
2. In a large wok or skillet, heat olive oil over medium-high heat. Add minced garlic and grated ginger, sautéing until fragrant.
3. Add the rice cauliflower to the wok, stirring constantly to cook evenly. Cook for 3-4 minutes until the cauliflower starts to soften.
4. Push the cauliflower rice to the side of the wok and add a bit more oil if needed. Add broccoli, carrots, bell pepper, and snap peas. Stir-fry the vegetables for 5-7 minutes until they are crisp-tender.
5. Combine the cooked protein of your choice with the vegetables and cauliflower rice.
6. Drizzle soy sauce or tamari and sesame oil over the mixture. Toss everything together until well combined and heated through.
7. Season with salt and pepper to taste.
8. Garnish the Cauliflower Rice Stir-Fry with chopped green onions and sesame seeds.
9. Serve hot and enjoy your low-carb, veggie-packed stir-fry.

Benefits:
- **Low in Carbs:** Cauliflower rice is a low-carb alternative to traditional rice, making

this stir-fry suitable for those watching their carb intake.

- **Packed with Vegetables:** The colorful array of vegetables provides essential vitamins, minerals, and fiber.
- **Versatile Protein Options:** Customize the stir-fry with your choice of protein to meet your dietary preferences.

Application:
- **Quick Weeknight Dinner:** Whip up this stir-fry for a quick and healthy weeknight dinner that's both satisfying and nutritious.
- **Meal Prep Option:** Prepare a large batch and portion it for convenient and healthy meal prep throughout the week.
- **Vegetarian Version:** Skip the meat and choose tofu or other plant-based proteins for a vegetarian-friendly option.

This Cauliflower Rice Stir-Fry is a creative and wholesome way to enjoy the flavors and textures of a classic stir-fry while incorporating the nutritional benefits of cauliflower.

It's a versatile dish that caters to various dietary preferences and makes for a delicious and satisfying meal.

Turkey and Quinoa Stuffed Peppers

Scenario:

Picture a colorful array of bell peppers filled with a hearty and nutritious mixture of lean ground turkey, quinoa, and vibrant vegetables.

These Turkey and Quinoa Stuffed Peppers are not only a feast for the eyes but also a wholesome and satisfying meal that's perfect for family dinners or entertaining guests.

Ingredients:

- 4 large bell peppers, halved and seeds removed
- 1 pound lean ground turkey
- 1 cup quinoa, cooked
- 1 onion, finely chopped
- 2 cloves garlic, minced
- 1 can (14 oz) diced tomatoes, drained
- 1 cup black beans, drained and rinsed
- 1 cup corn kernels (fresh or frozen)
- 1 teaspoon ground cumin
- 1 teaspoon chili powder
- Salt and pepper to taste
- 1 cup shredded cheese (cheddar, Monterey Jack, or your choice)
- Fresh cilantro or parsley for garnish

Preparation:

1. Preheat the oven to 375°F (190°C).
2. In a skillet, cook the ground turkey over medium heat until browned. Drain any excess fat.
3. Add chopped onions and minced garlic to the skillet. Sauté until the onions are translucent.
4. In a large bowl, combine the cooked turkey, quinoa, diced tomatoes, black beans, corn, ground cumin, chili powder, salt, and pepper. Mix well.
5. Arrange the halved bell peppers in a baking dish.
6. Spoon the turkey and quinoa mixture into each pepper half, pressing down gently to pack the filling.
7. Top each stuffed pepper with shredded cheese.
8. Cover the baking dish with foil and bake for 25-30 minutes. Remove the foil and bake for an additional 10-15 minutes or until the cheese is melted and bubbly.
9. Garnish with fresh cilantro or parsley before serving.

Benefits:

- **Lean Protein:** Turkey provides a lean source of protein essential for muscle health.

- **Whole Grain Goodness:** Quinoa is a complete protein and a good source of fiber.
- **Colorful Vegetables:** Bell peppers, tomatoes, black beans, and corn contribute a variety of vitamins, minerals, and antioxidants.

Application:
- **Family Dinner Favorite:** Serve these stuffed peppers as a wholesome and colorful family dinner option.
- **Make-Ahead Meal:** Prepare the filling in advance and assemble the stuffed peppers just before baking for a convenient make-ahead meal.
- **Party Entree:** Impress your guests by serving these Turkey and Quinoa Stuffed Peppers as a main course at gatherings or potluck dinners.

These Turkey and Quinoa Stuffed Peppers are a nutritious and flavorful way to enjoy a classic dish with a healthy twist. Packed with protein, whole grains, and vegetables, they make for a satisfying and well-balanced meal.

Mushroom and Spinach Omelet

Scenario:

Imagine starting your day with a wholesome and savory breakfast that combines earthy mushrooms, tender spinach, and fluffy eggs.

This Mushroom and Spinach Omelet is a delicious and nutritious way to kickstart your morning, providing a burst of energy and essential nutrients.

Ingredients:

- 3 large eggs
- 1 cup mushrooms, sliced
- 1 cup fresh spinach, chopped
- 1/2 onion, finely chopped
- 1 clove garlic, minced
- 1 tablespoon olive oil
- Salt and pepper to taste
- 1/4 cup shredded cheese (cheddar, feta, or your choice)
- Fresh herbs (parsley, chives) for garnish

Preparation:

1. In a non-stick skillet, heat olive oil over medium heat.
2. Add chopped onions and cook until softened, then add minced garlic and sauté for an additional minute.

3. Add sliced mushrooms to the skillet and cook until they release their moisture and become golden brown.
4. Stir in chopped spinach and cook until wilted. Season the mixture with salt and pepper to taste.
5. In a bowl, beat the eggs and season with a pinch of salt.
6. Push the vegetables to one side of the skillet, ensuring an even layer of the mixture.
7. Pour the beaten eggs into the empty side of the skillet. Let them set for a moment.
8. Using a spatula, gently lift the edges of the set eggs, allowing the uncooked eggs to flow underneath.
9. Once the eggs are mostly set, spoon the mushroom and spinach mixture onto one half of the omelet.
10. Sprinkle shredded cheese over the filling.
11. Fold the other half of the omelet over the filling, creating a half-moon shape.
12. Cook for another minute until the cheese melts, and the eggs are cooked through.
13. Slide the omelet onto a plate, garnish with fresh herbs, and serve hot.

Benefits:
- **Protein-Rich:** Eggs provide a high-quality source of protein, essential for muscle health.
- **Iron and Vitamins:** Spinach is rich in iron, while mushrooms provide essential vitamins and minerals.
- **Healthy Fats:** Olive oil contributes heart-healthy monounsaturated fats.

Application:
- **Breakfast Boost:** Enjoy this omelet as a filling and nutritious breakfast to start your day right.
- **Brunch Delight:** Serve the Mushroom and Spinach Omelet at brunch gatherings for a crowd-pleasing option.
- **Quick Dinner Option:** Whip up this omelet for a quick and light dinner on busy evenings.

This Mushroom and Spinach Omelet is a versatile and satisfying dish that combines the earthiness of mushrooms, the freshness of spinach, and the richness of eggs.

Whether enjoyed for breakfast, brunch, or dinner, it's a delightful way to incorporate a variety of flavors and nutrients into your meals.

Salmon and Asparagus Foil Packets

Scenario:
Visualize a hassle-free and delicious dinner where the flavors of succulent salmon and vibrant asparagus meld together in a perfect symphony.

These Salmon and Asparagus Foil Packets are not only easy to prepare but also ensure a flavorful and healthy meal that's ready in no time.

Ingredients:
- 4 salmon fillets
- 1 bunch asparagus, trimmed
- 1 lemon, thinly sliced
- 4 cloves garlic, minced
- 2 tablespoons fresh dill, chopped
- 2 tablespoons olive oil
- Salt and pepper to taste
- Optional: Red pepper flakes for a touch of heat

Preparation:
1. Preheat the oven to 400°F (200°C).
2. Cut four large pieces of aluminum foil, each large enough to wrap a salmon fillet and asparagus.

3. Place a salmon fillet in the center of each foil piece.
4. Arrange asparagus around each salmon fillet.
5. Drizzle olive oil over each salmon fillet and asparagus bundle.
6. Sprinkle minced garlic and chopped fresh dill over the salmon and asparagus.
7. Season with salt and pepper to taste. Add red pepper flakes if you desire a bit of heat.
8. Place lemon slices on top of each salmon fillet.
9. Fold the foil over the salmon and asparagus, sealing the edges to create a packet.
10. Place the foil packets on a baking sheet and bake in the preheated oven for 15-20 minutes, or until the salmon is cooked through and flakes easily.
11. Carefully open the foil packets, garnish with additional dill if desired, and serve hot.

Benefits:

- **Omega-3 Fatty Acids:** Salmon is a rich source of omega-3 fatty acids, promoting heart and brain health.
- **Vitamins and Antioxidants:** Asparagus is packed with vitamins A, C, and K, as well as antioxidants.

- **Anti-Inflammatory Herbs:** Fresh dill not only adds flavor but also provides anti-inflammatory properties.

Application:
- **Weeknight Dinner:** These foil packets make for a quick and convenient weeknight dinner option.
- **Outdoor Grilling:** Prepare the packets and cook them on the grill for a delightful outdoor meal.
- **Entertaining Guests:** Impress your guests by serving individual foil packets, allowing for an elegant presentation.

These Salmon and Asparagus Foil Packets are a foolproof way to achieve a flavorful and nutritious meal with minimal effort and cleanup.

The foil packets lock in the juices and flavors, resulting in moist and perfectly cooked salmon paired with tender asparagus. Enjoy a stress-free dinner that's both delicious and health-conscious.

Vegetarian Stir-Fry

Scenario:
Envision a vibrant and flavorful stir-fry that celebrates the goodness of a variety of colorful vegetables. This Vegetarian Stir-Fry is a quick and versatile dish that brings together the crunchiness of fresh vegetables with the savory notes of a delicious stir-fry sauce, creating a satisfying and wholesome meal.

Ingredients:
- 1 cup broccoli florets
- 1 bell pepper (any color), thinly sliced
- 1 carrot, julienned
- 1 cup snap peas, trimmed
- 1 cup mushrooms, sliced
- 1 cup firm tofu, cubed
- 3 tablespoons soy sauce or tamari
- 1 tablespoon hoisin sauce
- 1 tablespoon sesame oil
- 1 tablespoon vegetable oil
- 2 cloves garlic, minced
- 1 tablespoon ginger, grated
- 2 green onions, sliced
- Sesame seeds for garnish
- Cooked rice or noodles for serving

Preparation:

1. In a small bowl, mix together soy sauce or tamari, hoisin sauce, and sesame oil to create the stir-fry sauce. Set aside.
2. Heat vegetable oil in a wok or large skillet over medium-high heat.
3. Add minced garlic and grated ginger to the hot oil, sautéing until fragrant.
4. Add cubed tofu to the wok and cook until golden brown on all sides. Remove tofu from the wok and set aside.
5. In the same wok, add more oil if needed. Stir-fry broccoli, bell pepper, carrot, snap peas, and mushrooms until they are crisp-tender.
6. Return the cooked tofu to the wok and pour the stir-fry sauce over the vegetables and tofu.
7. Toss everything together until the vegetables and tofu are evenly coated with the sauce.
8. Add sliced green onions and toss for an additional minute.
9. Serve the Vegetarian Stir-Fry over cooked rice or noodles.
10. Garnish with sesame seeds and additional green onions.

Benefits:
- **Plant-Powered Protein:** Tofu is an excellent source of plant-based protein, essential for muscle health.
- **Fiber and Vitamins:** A variety of vegetables provide fiber, vitamins, and minerals for overall well-being.
- **Healthy Fats:** Sesame oil contributes heart-healthy monounsaturated fats.

Application:
- **Quick Weeknight Dinner:** This Vegetarian Stir-Fry is a perfect go-to option for a quick and nutritious weeknight dinner.
- **Meatless Monday Dish:** Incorporate this stir-fry into your Meatless Monday routine for a satisfying and plant-powered meal.
- **Meal Prep Favorite:** Make a large batch and divide it into containers for convenient and healthy meal prep throughout the week.

This Vegetarian Stir-Fry is not only a feast for the eyes but also a celebration of the delicious and nutritious possibilities of plant-based ingredients. Enjoy the variety of textures and flavors in every bite.

Grilled Chicken and Quinoa Bowl

Scenario:

Visualize a wholesome and satisfying meal where grilled chicken, nutty quinoa, and a colorful assortment of fresh vegetables come together in a nourishing bowl.

This Grilled Chicken and Quinoa Bowl is not only a feast for your taste buds but also a balanced and nutritious option for a well-rounded meal.

Ingredients:

- 1-pound boneless, skinless chicken breasts
- 1 cup quinoa, rinsed
- 2 cups mixed vegetables (bell peppers, cherry tomatoes, zucchini, etc.), diced
- 1 avocado, sliced
- 1/4 cup fresh cilantro, chopped
- 2 tablespoons olive oil
- Juice of 1 lemon
- 2 cloves garlic, minced
- 1 teaspoon dried oregano
- Salt and pepper to taste

Preparation:

1. Preheat the grill to medium-high heat.

2. Season the chicken breasts with olive oil, lemon juice, minced garlic, dried oregano, salt, and pepper.
3. Grill the chicken breasts for 6-8 minutes per side or until fully cooked and grill marks appear. Allow them to rest for a few minutes before slicing.
4. While the chicken is grilling, cook quinoa according to package instructions. Fluff with a fork once cooked.
5. In a large bowl, mix the cooked quinoa with diced mixed vegetables.
6. Assemble the bowls by placing a portion of quinoa and vegetable mixture in each bowl.
7. Top with sliced grilled chicken.
8. Garnish with avocado slices and chopped cilantro.
9. Drizzle with additional olive oil and lemon juice if desired.
10. Season with salt and pepper to taste.

Benefits:
- **High-Quality Protein:** Grilled chicken is a lean source of high-quality protein essential for muscle health.
- **Whole Grain Goodness:** Quinoa is a complete protein and a good source of fiber.

- **Nutrient-Rich Vegetables:** Mixed vegetables provide a variety of vitamins, minerals, and antioxidants.
- **Healthy Fats:** Avocado contributes heart-healthy monounsaturated fats.

Application:

- **Healthy Lunch Option:** Enjoy this Grilled Chicken and Quinoa Bowl as a satisfying and nutritious lunch.
- **Dinner for Two:** Prepare a romantic dinner by serving these bowls with a side salad and your favorite dressing.
- **Meal Prep Staple:** Make a batch for meal prep, dividing it into containers for easy and healthy lunches throughout the week.

This Grilled Chicken and Quinoa Bowl is a delightful combination of flavors and textures, offering a well-balanced and nutritious meal that's both satisfying and delicious. Customize the bowl with your favorite vegetables and herbs to suit your preferences.

Avocado and Egg Salad

Scenario:
Imagine a creamy and flavorful salad that combines the richness of ripe avocados with the protein-packed goodness of boiled eggs.

This Avocado and Egg Salad is not only a delightful twist on a classic, but it's also a quick and nutritious option for a light meal or refreshing side dish.

Ingredients:
- 2 ripe avocados, diced
- 4 hard-boiled eggs, chopped
- 1/4 cup red onion, finely chopped
- 1/4 cup fresh cilantro, chopped
- Juice of 1 lime
- 2 tablespoons mayonnaise
- Salt and pepper to taste
- Optional: Chili powder or paprika for a hint of spice
- Optional: Sliced cherry tomatoes for garnish

Preparation:
1. In a large bowl, combine diced avocados, chopped hard-boiled eggs, finely chopped red onion, and fresh cilantro.
2. In a small bowl, whisk together lime juice and mayonnaise.

3. Pour the lime and mayonnaise dressing over the avocado and egg mixture.
4. Gently toss the ingredients together until well combined.
5. Season with salt and pepper to taste. Add chili powder or paprika for a touch of spice if desired.
6. Garnish with sliced cherry tomatoes for a burst of color.
7. Refrigerate for 15-20 minutes to allow the flavors to meld.
8. Serve the Avocado and Egg Salad chilled, either on its own, as a side dish, or in a sandwich.

Benefits:
- **Healthy Fats:** Avocados are rich in monounsaturated fats, promoting heart health.
- **Protein-Packed:** Eggs provide high-quality protein essential for muscle health.
- **Vitamins and Minerals:** Cilantro and lime contribute vitamins and minerals, enhancing the nutritional profile of the salad.

Application:
- **Light Lunch Option:** Enjoy this Avocado and Egg Salad as a satisfying and light lunch on its own.

- **Sandwich Filling:** Spread the salad between slices of whole-grain bread for a creamy and delicious sandwich.
- **Summer Picnic Dish:** Pack individual portions for a refreshing salad to enjoy at picnics or outdoor gatherings.

This Avocado and Egg Salad is a delightful blend of creamy, savory, and tangy flavors. It's a versatile dish that can be enjoyed in various ways, making it a go-to option for quick and nutritious meals.

Green Smoothie Bowl

Scenario:

Imagine starting your day with a vibrant and nutrient-packed bowl that not only nourishes your body but also delights your taste buds.

This Green Smoothie Bowl is a refreshing and wholesome option that combines the goodness of leafy greens, fruits, and nutritious toppings, creating a bowl full of energy and vitality.

Ingredients:

For the Smoothie Base:
- 2 cups fresh spinach or kale, washed
- 1 frozen banana, sliced
- 1/2 cup frozen pineapple chunks
- 1/2 avocado
- 1 cup unsweetened almond milk or your choice of milk
- 1 tablespoon chia seeds (optional for added thickness)
- Ice cubes (optional)

For Toppings:
- Sliced kiwi
- Fresh berries (blueberries, strawberries, raspberries)
- Granola
- Shredded coconut
- Chia seeds
- Drizzle of honey or maple syrup (optional)

Preparation:
1. In a blender, combine fresh spinach or kale, frozen banana slices, frozen pineapple chunks, avocado, almond milk, and chia seeds.
2. Blend until smooth and creamy. Add ice cubes if you prefer a colder and thicker consistency.
3. Pour the green smoothie into a bowl.
4. Arrange toppings on the smoothie base. Feel free to get creative with the arrangement.
5. Drizzle with honey or maple syrup for added sweetness if desired.
6. Serve the Green Smoothie Bowl immediately and enjoy with a spoon.

Benefits:
- **Leafy Greens for Nutrients:** Spinach or kale provides a rich source of vitamins, minerals, and antioxidants.
- **Fruits for Natural Sweetness:** Banana, pineapple, and avocado add natural sweetness and essential nutrients.
- **Healthy Fats:** Avocado contributes monounsaturated fats, promoting heart health.
- **Protein and Fiber:** Chia seeds offer a boost of protein and fiber for sustained energy.

Application:

- **Healthy Breakfast Option:** Start your day with this Green Smoothie Bowl for a nutrient-packed and energizing breakfast.
- **Post-Workout Refuel:** Enjoy as a refreshing and replenishing post-workout snack.
- **Customizable Snack:** Customize the toppings based on your preferences and dietary needs.

CONCLUSION

"As we near the end of this culinary journey with 'Fast Feast Repeat,' we find ourselves not at an endpoint, but rather at the start of a transformative lifestyle." We've gone beyond the ordinary in this cookbook, embracing the power of Intermittent Fasting, relishing tasty food, and creating a sustainable approach to well-being.

We've discovered not only a weight-loss approach, but a philosophy that applies to every area of our life, in the art of fasting and feasting. It's a voyage of self-discovery, with each dish proving the balance of nourishment and enjoyment.

As we say goodbye, may these pages serve as a continual reminder that our health is a never-ending tale, where every fast is an opportunity for regeneration and every feast is a celebration of vitality.

May the concepts of 'Fast Feast Repeat' reverberate in your kitchens, filling you with the joy of conscious living, the satisfaction of balanced nourishment, and the empowerment of a better, happier self.

Here's to a life well-feasted and wonderfully repeated—a voyage in which health and flavor dance in unison, producing a symphony that reverberates far beyond the kitchen.

Until we meet again, may each meal serve as a reminder of your great ability to mold your own well-being.
Happy fasting, joyous feasting, and a life magnificently repeated.